Contents

What Is Blood Type Diet?

The blood type diet is a fad diet sometimes used in alternative medicine to promote weight loss and fight disease. Alternative medicine typically aims to recognize an individual's biochemical uniqueness and tailor treatment accordingly. The blood type diet is based on the theory that your blood type determines the foods you should consume in order to achieve optimal health.

The diet plan was developed by Peter D'Adamo, a naturopathic physician who theorizes that people respond to various foods depending on their blood type.

The four different blood types are one marker that can theoretically be used to determine the right diet for your health and vitality. The idea behind the diet is that eating foods with lectins (a type of protein) that are incompatible with a person's blood type can cause blood cell clumping, called agglutination, and result in health problems such as heart or kidney disease or cancer. However, there is a lack of scientific evidence to support these claims.

D'Adamo also believes that a person's blood type affects their ability to digest various foods due to differences in digestive secretions associated with the different blood types. People who are type O, for example, are thought to digest meat well due to high levels of stomach acid.

D'Adamo suggests that by following a meal plan designed for your specific blood type, you can digest food with greater efficiency, avoid the negative effects of certain lectins, and—in turn—lose weight and enhance your overall health.

How Does the Blood Type Diet Work?

D'Adamo says that protein components in food called lectins bind with antigens on blood cells and lead to blood cell clumping, or agglutination. Avoiding agglutination, D'Adamo argues, can improve health by helping people manage weight better and fight cancer and heart disease.

Liz Weinandy, RD, at Ohio State University Wexner Medical Center in Columbus, Ohio, says that lectins can be dangerous to our health if eaten in large amounts, but the way D'Adamo presents their effects may be misleading. Reducing their potential health harms is relatively easy: For example, lectins found in beans can be eliminated simply by soaking the beans in water for a few hours and then boiling them for 10 minutes, Weinandy says.

But D'Adamo uses his theory to develop separate diets for people with blood types A, B, AB, and O. In addition, he recommends exercise and overall healthy habits, like drinking enough water, Weinandy explains. However, the diet is specific about which foods groups are allowed for different blood types — and that can be be restrictive, Weinandy says.

In fact, while people often have different nutritional needs, humans are complex animals, and chalking up these specifics to blood type may oversimplify those needs, Weinandy says.

"To base a whole diet on that is probably not very sensible

What You Need to Know

There is no specific timing for meals or fasting periods required on the blood type diet. However, the plan advises against drinking water or other beverages with meals because it will dilute the natural digestive enzymes and make it more difficult to digest foods.

What To Eat?

The blood type diet emphasizes certain foods and exercise plans for different blood types. Regardless of blood type, the diet emphasizes eating whole foods and minimizing the intake of processed foods. Here's a closer look at the prescribed plans:

- Type A: According to D'Adamo, people with type A blood are predisposed to heart disease, cancer, and diabetes, and do better on an organic, vegetarian diet with calming, centering exercise, such as yoga and tai chi.

- Type B: People with type B blood, according to D'Adamo, have a robust immune system and a tolerant digestive system, and are more adaptable than other blood types. He recommends moderate physical exercise and balance exercises, along with a "well-rounded" diet. According to the theory behind the diet, people with type B, however, are more susceptible to autoimmune disorders, such as chronic fatigue, lupus, and multiple sclerosis.

- Type AB: People with type AB blood are more biologically complex than other types, according to D'Adamo. Based on this belief, these people supposedly do best with a combination of the exercises and diets for types A and B, though meat should be limited. It is believed that this blood type tends to have lower rates of allergies, but heart disease, cancer, and anemia are common.

- Type O: Based on the blood type diet theory, people with type O blood do best with intense physical exercise and animal proteins, while dairy products and grains may cause problems. According to D'Adamo, gluten, lentils, kidney beans, corn, and cabbage can lead to weight gain in people with this blood type. Health conditions associated with type O include asthma, hay fever, and other allergies, and arthritis.

Compliant Foods

- Type A: Mostly vegetarian including fruits, vegetables, grains, beans, legumes, nuts, and seeds

- Type B: Highly varied diet—fruits, vegetables, grains, beans, legumes, meat, poultry, fish, eggs, and dairy

- Type AB: Mainly vegan, but any foods recommended for A or B types may be consumed

• Type O: Meat with a moderate amount of vegetables, eggs, nuts, and seeds

Non- Complaint Food

• Type A: Meat and dairy

• Type B: Nuts and seeds

• Type AB: No specific foods to avoid

• Type O: Dairy and grains

• People with blood type A, who D'Adamo calls the "cultivator," should follow a dairy-free, primarily vegetarian diet with a high intake of fruits, vegetables, grains, beans, legumes, and nuts and seeds.

• People with blood type B, who D'Adamo calls "the nomad," should eat a highly varied diet including fruits and vegetables, grains, beans, legumes, meat, poultry, fish, eggs, and dairy, but avoid intake of nuts and seeds.

• People with blood type AB, who D'Adamo calls "the enigma," can consume any food recommended for blood types A and B, although aiming for a mainly vegan diet is advised for this type.

• People with blood type O, who D'Adamo calls "the hunter," should stick to a dairy-free and grain-free diet high in meat, low in grains, and with a moderate amount of vegetables, eggs, nuts, and seeds.

In addition to specific foods, D'Adamo recommends different supplements for each blood type, which are available on his book's website. There is a specially formulated multivitamin, multimineral, lectin blocker, and probiotic/prebiotic blend for each blood type.

Benefits

The blood type diet encourages exercise. Research shows that regular exercise combined with a healthy diet can lead to weight loss and promote weight management. However, there is no research to support the blood type diet as an effective weight-loss strategy.

Each blood type plan emphasizes choosing whole foods. The program also offers a wide variety of compliant foods for some of the blood types, which may make it easier to stick with.

Although each blood type comes with its own set of dietary restrictions, the program is not a low-calorie diet with unhealthy restrictions on calorie intake. Plans for types B and AB are more well-rounded and can provide most if not all of the necessary nutrients for a well-balanced diet. However, the plans for types A and O restrict certain healthy food groups, which is not a smart long-term eating plan for many people.

Drawbacks

Eating for your specific blood type is not rooted in science. The available research on the blood type diet includes a study published in the journal PLoS One in 2014. For the study, 1,455 participants filled out questionnaires designed to determine how frequently they'd consumed certain foods during a one-month period.

In their analysis of the questionnaires, researchers found that following a diet similar to the diet prescribed for blood type A or blood type AB was associated with lower blood pressure and lower cholesterol levels.

Following a diet similar to the diet prescribed for blood type O was associated with lower levels of triglycerides (high levels of this blood fat have been associated with an increased risk of cardiovascular disease), while no significant association was found for the blood type B diet.

Is the Blood Type Diet a Healthy?

Depending on your blood type, this plan may or may not meet the USDA's definition of a healthy meal plan.

- The Type AB diet is the least restrictive and allows for the widest variety of foods to ensure adequate nutrition.

• The Type A diet prohibits meat and dairy, which have nutrients, namely protein, that can be found in other foods with careful planning.

• The Type B diet also offers a varied diet, with the exception of nuts and seeds, and meets most of the requirements of the USDA healthy eating plan.

• The Type O diet avoids dairy and grains, which are considered important parts of a healthy diet, according to the USDA. With careful planning, however, the nutrients found in grains and dairy can be made up by eating a variety of vegetables.

Blood Type Dietary Recommendation

According to D'Adamo, those with the following blood types should follow these dietary recommendations:

Type O: The hunter – has better overall health when eating a lean protein diet (meat, fish, poultry, certain fruits and vegetables) with less dairy, legumes, and grains; D'Adamo believes gluten is a leading cause for weight gain in this blood type.

Type A: The cultivator – has a more sensitive immune system and has an increased risk of developing heart disease, cancer, and diabetes. These people should consume a fresh and organic vegetarian diet.

Type B: The nomad – has a strong immune system as well as a tolerant digestive system and survives chronic diseases better than other blood types. These people should consume both plants and meats (except chicken and pork), and can also have some dairy. However, they should avoid wheat, corn, lentils, tomatoes, and a few other foods.

Type AB: The enigma- the newest blood type in terms of evolution and the most complex. Seafood, tofu, dairy, beans, and grains are a large part of the recommended diet for this group. They should avoid corn, beef, chicken, and kidney beans.

This sounds like healthy eating, right? True. There are many aspects of these ways of eating that have significant nutrition improvements compared to the average Western Diet high in processed foods, added sugars, and unhealthy fats. But that doesn't mean that there is any truth behind the idea that your blood type affects your body's interactions with foods.

Lectins are a Proposed Link Between Diet and Blood Type

One of the central theories of the blood type diet has to do with proteins called lectins.

Lectins are a diverse family of proteins that can bind sugar molecules.

These substances are considered to be antinutrients, and may have negative effects on the lining of the gut.

According to the blood type diet theory, there are many lectins in the diet that specifically target different ABO blood types.

It is claimed that eating the wrong types of lectins could lead to agglutination (clumping together) of red blood cells.

There is actually evidence that a small percentage of lectins in raw, uncooked legumes, can have agglutinating activity specific to a certain blood type.

For example, raw lima beans may interact only with the red blood cells in people with blood type A.

Overall, however, it appears that the majority of agglutinating lectins react with all ABO blood types.

In other words, lectins in the diet are NOT blood-type specific, with the exception of a few varieties of raw legumes.

This may not even have any real-world relevance, because most legumes are soaked and/or cooked before consumption, which destroys the harmful lectins.

Is There Any Scientific Evidence Behind The Blood Type Diet?

Research on ABO blood types has advanced rapidly in the past few years and decades.

There is now strong evidence that people with certain blood types can have a higher or lower risk of some diseases.

For example, type Os have a lower risk of heart disease, but a higher risk of stomach ulcers.

However, there are no studies showing this to have anything to do with diet.

In a large observational study of 1,455 young adults, eating a type A diet (lots of fruits and vegetables) was associated with better health markers. But this effect was seen in everyone following the type A diet, not just individuals with type A blood.

In a major 2013 review study where researchers examined the data from over a thousand studies, they did not find a single well-designed study looking at the health effects of the blood type diet.

They concluded: "No evidence currently exists to validate the purported health benefits of blood type diets."

Of the 4 studies identified that somewhat related to ABO blood type diets, they were all poorly designed.

One of the studies that found a relationship between blood types and food allergies actually contradicted the blood type diet's recommendations.

Can the Blood Type Diet Help People With Certain Conditions?

But there is some evidence that people with certain blood types may be more prone to certain illnesses. For instance, individuals with type O blood may be at a greater risk for duodenal ulcers. Those who are type A may be at an increased risk for atrophic gastritis. Some blood type O patients have specific proteins that are attacked by the bacteria Helicobacter pylori, which is commonly linked to ulcers.

Similarly, that bacteria has also been associated with atrophic gastritis, though the exact relationship between type A blood and atrophic gastritis is not known.

But there's no evidence to support the theory that eating a diet tailored to a certain blood type has any effect on these conditions.

Is the Blood Type Diet Safe? What to Expect If You Try It

There's concern that the Eat Right fpr your blood Type diet for those with blood type O is too protein heavy. Animal protein, especially red meat, has been linked to health problems, such as heart disease and colorectal cancer.

Also, dietitians say it's possible that individuals may experience nutritional deficiencies when following the eating plan.

The diet recommends calcium supplements for [type O and type A individuals] who can't eat dairy, for example. "But you can only absorb a certain amount of calcium from supplements, and you get so much more from food. If you follow this diet for a long time, you could experience vitamin and mineral deficiencies."

Another potential long-term problem with the blood type diet is a drawback common to many diets: Restriction leads to boredom. When you take away favorite foods, it's almost a death knell for any dietary program, whether there is solid advice or not. If you tell people to avoid fruit or anything made with white flour, they can go back to those foods with a vengeance later on. Some critics argue that Eat Right 4 Your Type places too much emphasis on blood type and fails to take into account individual differences. "I would look at an individual's food preferences and health challenges, such as stroke risk, hypertension, and allergies,".

Should You Try the Blood Type Diet for Weight Loss and Health Improvements?

Whatever you do to lose weight, it has to be reasonable to be sustainable. The blood type diet may work for some people, but given how restrictive it is, people may have trouble sticking with it long term — and thus not be able to keep off the weight they lost.

Still, for people curious about the benefits of the blood type diet, There is no harm in trying it for a short period of time. "More important, make sure that you are eating wholesome foods that are not processed," she advises, noting that she often directs patients more toward a

Mediterranean diet or a DASH diet for overall health and weight loss.

Health Benefits

Proponents of the blood type diet claim that the program can help you burn fat more efficiently, increase your energy levels, support your immune system, and lower your risk of major health problems like heart disease and cancer. However, there is currently a lack of scientific evidence to support these claims.

In addition, there is no research to support that the blood-type diet is an effective weight-loss strategy.

Health Risks

Although proponents of the blood type diet suggest that the use of dietary supplements can help people following the diet plan meet their nutritional needs, such supplements are not regarded as a reasonable substitute for a healthy, balanced meal plan.

Since the diets prescribed for blood types A and O are restrictive, there's some concern that individuals following these diets may fail to achieve sufficient intake of many vitamins and minerals that are essential for health.

In addition, a research review published in 2013 found that further studies are still needed to support any of the health claims associated with the blood type diet. In this review, scientists looked at 16 previously published reports on the blood type diet and concluded that "no evidence currently exists to validate the purported health benefits of blood type diets."

Blood Type Diet Sample Menu for Each Blood Type

Here is a sample one-day diet for each blood type, based on D'Adamo's recommended recipes:

Type O

- Breakfast: Two slices of organic bread with almond butter, vegetable juice, and a banana
- Lunch: A spinach salad with roast beef and fruit slices

- Snack: Fruit
- Dinner: Lamb stew with a variety of vegetables
- Dessert: Fruit salad

Type A

- Breakfast: Buckwheat pancakes topped with maple syrup, tahini, jam, or lemon juice
- Lunch: Curried peanut tempeh with carrots, celery, and broccoli
- Snack: Trail mix
- Dinner: Rice pasta with feta and greens
- Dessert: Crumb apple pie

Type B

- Breakfast: Oatmeal with unsalted butter or ghee

- Lunch: Indian curry salad
- Snack: Kale chips
- Dinner: Apple-braised lamb shoulder chops
- Dessert: Carob fudge

Type AB

- Breakfast: Silken tofu scramble with carrots and zucchini
- Lunch: Cream of mushroom soup
- Snack: White bean hummus with celery sticks
- Dinner: Grilled cod and veggies over apricot-walnut couscous
- Dessert: Flourless almond butter and raisin cookies

BLOOD TYPE DIET RECIPES

The following recipes are blood type-friendly while also being a treat to the taste buds. Try some of these blood type diet recipes today.

Egg and Seaweed Soup

Prepartion time

30 minutes

Ingredient

- 2 cups turkey stock
- 2 cups water
- 1/2 cup sliced vegetable of choice (celery, carrots, mushrooms, etc.)
- 1 teaspoon arrowroot

- 2 sheets of dried Nori
- 1 egg
- dash of sea salt to taste
- 1 other teaspoon arrowroot
- 3 sprigs of green onion
- 2 teaspoon ume plum vinegar (or soy sauce)
- 1/4 tsp white pepper (optional)
- 1/4 tsp (or more) ground red pepper flakes (optional)
- 1/4 tsp marmite (optional)

Instructions

1. Boil the water and broth in a saucepan.

2. Add the vegetable and boil until crisp/tender.

3. Mix the arrowroot with a little water and pour into boiling soup to thicken.

4. Break up the Nori Seaweed sheets into small pieces and put into the soup mixture.

5. Mix the remaining tsp arrowroot with a little water, add the egg, and beat.

6. Turn off the heat until the top is calm, and slowly pour the egg mixture in thin threads, into the soup. Let sit for one minute, then bring to a gentle boil and stir gently to distribute eggs.

7. Add salt and spices, marmite, vinegar, etc. to taste and sprinkle with thinly sliced spring onions.

Spinach Feta Rice

Prepartion time

35 minutes

Ingredient

- 1 cup uncooked long-grain rice
- 1 cup fat-free chicken broth [Type B should sub]
- 1 cup water
- 1 medium onion, chopped
- 1 cup sliced portabello mushrooms (about 4 oz, or 4 big ones)
- 2 cloves garlic, minced
- 1 Tablespoon lemon juice

- 1/2 teaspoon salt
- 1/2 teaspoon dried oregano leaves, crushed
- 1 package chopped frozen spinach, cooked according to directions, then drained and pressed until most of water is gone. May use 6 cups shredded fresh spinach leaves instead
- 4 oz. feta cheese, crumbled

Instructions

1. Combine rice, broth, and water in medium saucepan.

2. Bring water to boil.

3. Add rice, stir once.

4. Reduce heat to low.

5. Cover and simmer 15-20 minutes (according to your package instructions) or until rice is tender and liquid is absorbed.

6. Cook and stir onion, mushrooms, and garlic in large skillet coated with nonstick cooking spray until onion is tender.

7. Add cooked spinach, oregano leaves, salt, and lemon juice so that it, too, is warm.

8. Add entire mixture to rice (or vice versa), add feta cheese, stir well and it's ready to serve.

Sesame salt

Prepartion time

15 minutes

Ingredient

- 3/4 cup sesame seeds
- 1 Tablespoon sea salt

Instructions

1. Toast sesame seeds in a dry pan until they become light brown and you smell a nutty aroma.

2. Take off heat and add sea salt.

3. Stir well.

4. Put in a blender or food processor and blend until smooth.

Marvelous Millet

Prepartion time

25 minutes

Ingredient

- 1 onion
- 2 carrots
- 3 tablespoons Olive Oil
- 1 cup millet
- 2 1/2 cups water
- 1 veggie bouillon (or un-chicken bouillon)
- 1/2 teaspoon Tumeric

Instructions

1. Chop onion.

2. Peel and dice carrots.

3. Saute the onion in olive oil in sauce pan until onion is soft and clear.

4. Add millet and sauté, stirring constantly, cover millet with oil and toast. Millet should be slightly brown.

5. Add water, bouillon, turmeric and bring to a boil.

6. Simmer for 15 minutes.

Basic Salad Dressing

Prepartion time

3 minutes

Ingredient

- 1/4 cup olive oil
- 1/4 cup lemon or lime juice
- 1/4 cup agave
- 1/4 teaspoon salt
- 1/4 teaspoon garlic powder
- 1/2 teaspoon onion powder

Instructions

1. Combine all ingredients in a resealable bottle.
2. Shake well before serving.

3. May be stored in the refrigerator for up to a week.

4. Shake before each use.

kid friendly grilled salmon on a stick!

Prepartion time

30 minutes

Ingredient

- One large salmon - ocean caught
- olive oil
- garlic powder
- sea salt

Instructions

1. Preheat grill, brush with olive oil.

2. Leave the skin on one side of the salmon. Cut into one inch strips.

3. Stick pieces on skewers. Wash hands and spice liberally.

4. Place skewers, meat side down, onto grill.

5. Do not flip too soon! Let the meat get nice and brown before flipping over.

6. On my gas stove top, I started the grill on 4 and then turned it down to 3.

Kate's Chicken Fingers

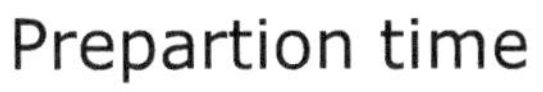

Prepartion time

30 minutes

Ingredient

- 10-12 chicken breast strips
- 1 egg
- 1 cup kamut or rice flour [or spelt flour]
- 1 teaspoon onion powder
- 1 teaspoon garlic powder
- 1 teaspoon freshly ground black peppercorns (optional)
- 1 teaspoon sea salt

- 1 cup ghee

Instructions

1. Break egg into bowl and whisk until combined.
2. Mix raw chicken into egg in bowl.
3. Combine dry ingredients and sprinkle one layer on a plate.
4. Remove chicken from egg (one strip at a time) and coat with flour mixture on plate.
5. Repeat until all strips are coated.
6. Heat large pan to medium.
7. Add half of the ghee to the pan and melt.

8. Place chicken strips in pan and fry for about 2-3 minutes per side, adding more ghee as necessary.

9. Remove chicken strips from pan and place onto a bed of paper towel to absorb any excess ghee.

Black Bean Soup with Meat

Prepartion time

1 hour 15 minutes

Ingredient :

- 1 Tablespoon Olive Oil

- 2 Onions Chopped
- 10 Cloves Garlic Minced
- 1 Pound Grass Fed Ground Beef
- 1 Package Applegate Roasted Red Pepper Sausage
- 3 teaspoon Chili Powder
- 2 teaspoon Cumin
- 5 cups Beef Broth
- 2 cans(15 Oz)Black Beans or 4 cups Prepared Black Beans
- 1/2 cup Wakame (Sea Vegetable)
- 3 cups Basmati Rice Precooked
- Sea Salt/Fresh Ground Green Peppercorns to Taste

Instructions

1. In a large frying pan, heat oil over medium heat; brown onions, garlic and sausage.

2. In a separate frying pan, brown ground beef, drain and add to onion mixture.

3. Continue cooking adding chili powder, cumin, beef broth, Wakame, and one can of the beans.

4. Meanwhile, in a food processor or blender, puree the remaining can of beans and add to the pan.

5. Reduce heat, cover and simmer for 15 - 20 minutes on medium.

6. Add rice, reduce heat to low and simmer for another 30 minutes.

Agave-Sweetened Lemonade

Prepartion time

2 minutes

Ingredients

- 1/2 Cup of freshly squeezed lemon juice
- 1/2 Cup of organic light agave syrup
- 1 quart of water
- a few lemon slices for garnish (optional)

Instructions

1. Mix everything together.

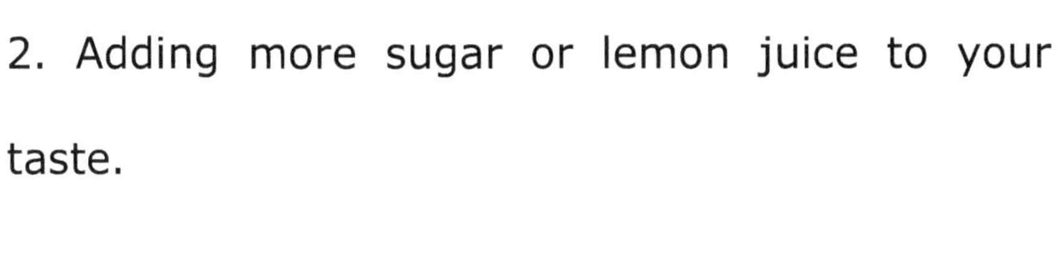
2. Adding more sugar or lemon juice to your taste.

Almond Toffee

Prepartion time

40 minutes

Ingredients

- 1/2 cup unsalted butter
- 1/2 cup agave nectar
- 1 Cup of chopped almonds

Instructions

1. prepare a tray with non stick cooking paper.

2. Melt the butter in a saucepan, over medium to low heat.

3. Stir in the agave nectar with a wooden spoon.

4. Continue to stir constantly until the mixture comes together and pulls away from the side of the pan. To test for doneness, have a cup of cold water standing by, and drop a bit of the mixture into the cold water.

5. It should turn hard immediately. But don't delay, because once it starts pulling away from the sides of the pan, it can burn quickly.

6. As soon as the mixture pulls away from the sides of the pan, add chopped almonds and stir, turn it out onto the non stick cooking paper.

7. Scrape the sides of the pan with the wooden spoon.

8. Allow to cool for about 20-30 minutes, then break/cut into irregular shapes of any size.

Tabouleh

Prepartion time

30 minutes

Ingredients

- Bulghur Wheat

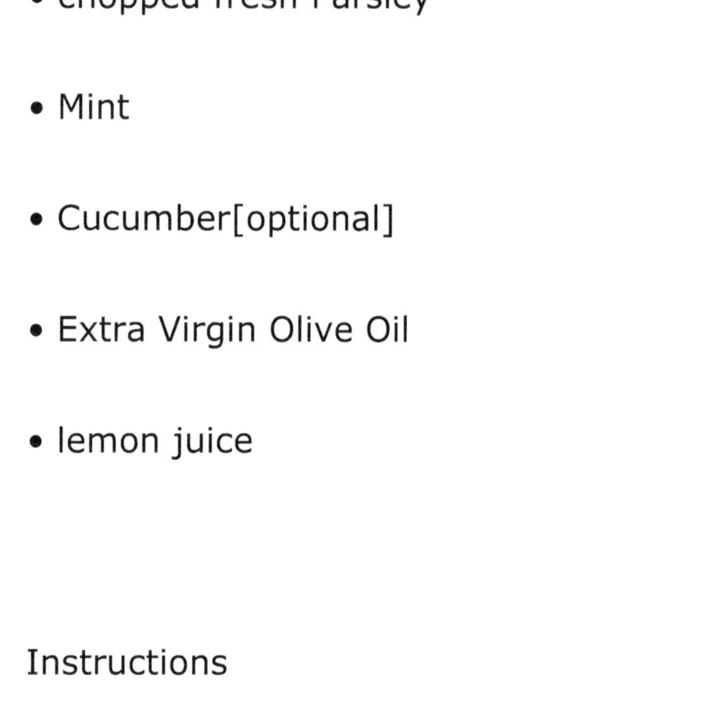

- chopped fresh Parsley
- Mint
- Cucumber[optional]
- Extra Virgin Olive Oil
- lemon juice

Instructions

1. Soak the wheat in boiling water and then drain

2. A selection of chopped fresh Parsley, Mint and Cucumber[optional] stirred through the wheat then dressed with Extra Virgin Olive Oil and lemon juice.

3. Allow to stand for at least one hour and it tastes better served at room temperature.

Lahmacun Recipe

Prepartion time

2 hours

Ingredients

For the dough:

- 1 teaspoon dry active yeast
- 1/2 teaspoon sugar
- 1+1/2 cup of warm water

- 4+1/2 cups of flour (you can use plain wheat)[or compliant]
- Little oil to brush the dough

For the topping:

- 12 ounces minced lamb
- 1 big onion
- 2-3 cloves of garlic
- 2 Tablespoon butter
- 1+1/2 cups fresh curly parsley
- 1 cup of fresh mint
- 1 medium tomato
- 1 teaspoon chili pepper

- 1 jalapeno (optional)
- 1 teaspoon paprika (optional)
- 1 teaspoon cumin (optional)
- salt, according to your own taste
- Juice of 1 lemon
- little oil to brush the dough

Instructions

For the dough:

1. In a small bowl mix yeast and the sugar.
2. Add 1/2 cup of warm water, stir well, close the lid (or cover with plate).
3. You can leave the bowl on the counter but I usually put it somewhere warm. Warmness

accelerates the process and better activates the yeast. Activating yeast is important to have a better rising dough.

4. Keep the mixture warm for about 15 minutes without opening the lid. When the time is up, you should have a nice foamy liquid. Even if you do not, still keep it and make the dough. It will still work.

5. In a large bowl combine the remaining water, flour and the yeast mixture.

6. Mix everything well and knead it into a nice soft, springy dough. It should be soft as your ear lobes.

7. Add flour or water, as needed.

8. A well-kneaded dough will be much easier to work with later. Keep this in mind!

9. Coat the dough with just a little bit of oil, cover with damp cloth and leave it to rise in a warm place. I usually cover the bowl with the lid and bundle it up nicely to have a good volume dough.

10. Give it a rest for around 1 hour before you take it out from the cover. When you do take the dough out, make sure it has doubled in size.

11. Once the time is up, open up the lid and punch the dough a little.

12. Flour the working surface and drop the dough.

13. Cut it into pieces smaller than a tennis ball but larger that a golf ball.

14. You should have about 10-12 pieces.

15. Roll each one and place on the floured surface.

16. Cover with a damp cloth and let it stand until your topping is ready (20 min).

17. Turn the oven on and keep it at 420 degrees Fahrenheit.

For the topping:

1. Meanwhile, prepare the topping. This picture really makes me smile. I love vegetables. I also love that ground beef in there :)

2. Wash the greens well and chop them nicely. I usually wash and soak parsley with mint in water prior to using them. This way all the dirt remains in the water.

3. Cut the onion and garlic in pieces, put the pieces into a chopper and chop until nicely minced.

4. Heat the skillet on medium-high, melt the butter, add onion+garlic mixture, saute for about 1 minute.

5. Reduce the heat to low, close the lid and simmer for 2 more minutes.

6. Take the skillet off the burner and cool the onion mixture.

7. Peel the skin off tomato and cut it to very small pieces. A lot of people like to seed the tomatoes. I don't like it, since it also removes all the juice from the tomato. But if you feel like seeding the tomato, go ahead.

8. Have all the ingredients in one big bowl. At this point, add chili pepper, salt, cumin, lemon juice, paprika, chopped jalapenos (or chopped pickled hot peppers) and mix everything very well. I am stressing this – the ingredients MUST be well mixed!

9. The dough is well rested at this point. Take one by one and roll into a round, flat circle or an oval measuring up to 5 mm in height. I like my Lahmacuns very thin. This way they come out a little crispy.

10. Some use pizza stones to bake Lahmacuns. While it is a good alternative for the original brick ovens, in my opinion, it is not very practical. So, I suggest using regular baking sheets.

11. Sprinkle some non-fat cooking spray (or just a little oil will work), place rolled dough on the sheet, slightly brush with some olive oil (canola oil works too) top up with 2 Tablespoons of the ready topping. Spread the topping evenly and very thinly.

12. I place 2 doughs in one regular 11″ x 17″ size baking sheet.

13. If you have bigger sheets and want to use those, you are more than welcome to do so. 3 baking sheets are enough to keep the whole process going pretty fast.

14. Put two baking sheets in the oven at a time. The top one usually gets baked faster. When you take the ready batch out, rotate the bottom one

to the top and place a new batch on the lower rack.

15. The oven should remain at 420F – not too high and not too low. Since you are going to be constantly opening the oven, the temperature ideally will stay at about 370F.

16. Cooked Lahmacuns are crispy at the ends and softer in the middle. Corners usually get nicely tanned. Take them off the baking sheet to a wider container and cover with a towel until you are done with every single one of them.

17. Humidity under the towel will soften Lahmacuns, making it very easy for you to roll them around the fresh ingredients you might want to use.

18. Pace yourself, the process is a little overwhelming. But the end result is worth every minute of your time in the kitchen. We really enjoy Lahmacuns rolled around onions, some fresh curly parsley and hand-squeezed lemon juice.

Pineapple, Carrot, Walnut and Raisin Cake

Prepartion time

50 minutes

Ingredients

- 1 1/3 cup spelt flour
- 1 2/3 cup sugar
- 2/3 cup kamut flour
- 1 cup oil or melted butter
- 2 teaspoon baking soda
- 2 cups grated carrots
- 1 + teaspoon sea salt
- 2 cups crushed pineapple
- 2 teaspoons cinnamon
- 1 cup raisins
- 4 eggs
- 1 cup chopped walnuts

Instructions

1. Sift together dry ingredients; set aside.

2. Mix eggs, sugar, and oil or melted butter, stirring well.

3. Add carrots, DRAINED pineapple, walnuts, and raisins; beat after each addition.

4. Add sifted ingredients; stir well.

5. Pour into greased and floured 9"x13" pan.

6. Bake at 350 degrees for 40 minutes.

Lamb Stew with Collard Greens

Prepartion time

1 hour

Ingredients

- 2 Tbsp compliant flour (rice, soy) seasoned with 1/8 tsp cayenne, 1/4 tsp ground black pepper and 1/2 tsp sea salt (cayenne could be omitted)
- 1 lb lean lamb, diced into 2 inch cubes
- 2 Tbsp olive oil
- 6 c vegetable stock
- 3 lg carrots, cut into 2 inch rounds
- 2 lg stalks celery, cut into 1 in pieces
- 3 cloves garlic, peeled and chopped

- 5 red new potatoes, washed but not peeled, cut into eighths (sweets, yams or parsnips could be used)
- 1 tsp dried rosemary
- 2 Tbsp minced parsley
- 5 lg collard green leaves, chopped

Instructions

1. Put seasoned flour in a plastic bag, add meat pieces and toss until coated.

2. Heat oil in the bottom of a stockpot.

3. On medium-high heat, lightly brown meat pieces about 1 minute on each side.

4. Add stock, carrots, celery, potatoes, garlic and rosemary.

5. Cover and bring to a boil.

6. Lower heat and simmer for 40 minutes.

7. Add parsley and collard greens and cook for 10 minutes more.

8. Season to taste with salt, pepper and cayenne

Japanese Salad Dressing

Prepartion time

5 minutes

Ingredients

- 1/2 cup olive oil (or 1 cup olive oil if omitting sesame oil)
- 1/2 cup sesame oil
- 1/3 cup fresh lemon (lime or kumquat)juice
- 2 large cloves garlic
- 2 Tbs peeled fresh ginger
- 3 Tbs sweet onion
- 2 medium carrots
- 1 tsp honey (optional)
- salt to taste

Instructions

1. Combine all ingredients at one time using a blender.

2. Enjoy!!!

Moroccan Lamb Sausage Patties from Food Network

Prepartion time

15 minutes

Ingredients

- Optional Yogurt Sauce (omit for Type O's):
- 1 cup plain yogurt (regular or nonfat)
- 2 tablespoons chopped fresh cilantro
- 1/2 teaspoon ground cumin

Sausage Patties:

- 1 pound ground lamb
- 2 cloves garlic, minced or pressed
- 2 Tablespoons chopped fresh cilantro
- 2 Tablespoons red wine vinegar (omit except for Type B's)
- 1 Tablespoon paprika (sweet or hot)
- 1-1/2 teaspoons sea salt
- 1 teaspoon ground cumin
- 1 teaspoon ground coriander
- 1/2 teaspoon ground allspice (B's and AB's can omit substitute w 1/8 teaspoon ground clove)
- Ground black pepper (A's and AB's omit)

Instructions

1. To prepare yogurt sauce (omit for Type O's): In a small bowl, mix yogurt, cilantro, and cumin.

2. Set aside.

3. To prepare sausage patties, put meat in a large bowl and add all blood type appropriate ingredients.

4. Mix with your hands until well blended.

5. Form mixture into 8 small patties.

6. Cook patties on a barbecue (or in a nonstick frying pan or well-oiled skillet) until seared on the outside and cooked through inside, about 8 minutes total.

7. Instant thermometer internal temperature reading of 165 degrees Fahrenheit.

8. Serve drizzled with optional yogurt sauce.

Power Smoothie

Prepartion time

5 minutes

Ingredients

- quarter a fresh pineapple
- handful of frozen berries
- splash of pineapple and/or apple juice
- equal amount of light soy milk and/or rice milk
- 2 Tablespoons of soy powder protein (found in HFS of supermarket)and/or silken tofu

- Scoop of frozen berry yogurt (optional)

Instructions

1. Put them all in the blender together and whirl until smooth like a thick shake.
2. yummy.

Grilled Tuna Steaks

Prepartion time

5 minutes

Ingredients

- 2 large tuna steaks

- 3/4 cup olive oil
- 1 Tablespoon tamari
- 1/4 cup chopped onion
- 1 Tablespoon lemon juice
- dash of garlic, onion, parsley and other compliant spice according to taste

Instructions

1. Add all ingredients except tuna in a large zip lock bag.
2. Once all ingredients are mixed together wash tuna well and add to bag.
3. Zip bag, remove any air, and marinate in frig for 1-2 hours.

4. Grill tuna approx 5-8 minutes depending on thickness of tuna on each side.

5. Any extra sauce add as grilling.

Carob Brownies

Prepartion time

30 minutes

Ingredients

- 15 teaspoons carob powder
- 1/3 cup ghee
- 1-1/2 cups sugar [or 3/4 cups agave nectar]
- 4 eggs

- 1 teaspoon vanilla [optional]
- 1-1/2 cups spelt flour
- less than 1 teaspoon baking soda [not in Typebase]
- less than 1 teaspoon salt
- 1 cup chopped walnuts or other nuts

Instructions

- Heat oven to 325F.
- Grease 9x13' baking pan.
- Melt Ghee and carob powder in medium saucepan over low heat.
- Remove from heat.
- Mix in sugar, eggs and vanilla.

- Stir in remaining ingredients.
- Spread in pan.
- Bake about 25 minutes or until brownies start to pull away from sides of pan.
- Do not overbake.
- Cool slightly.
- Cut into bars.

Harvest Fruit Salad

Prepartion time

10 minutes

Ingredients

- 2-3 apples (Granny Smith for tart, Fuji or Braeburn for sweet - or mixed for variety)
- 1/4 cup chopped pecans
- 1/4 cup shredded coconut
- 1/4 cup golden raisins
- 1/3 cup mini-marshmallows [check ingredients]
- 1 cup low fat vanilla yogurt

Instructions

1. Dice apples into bite sized pieces, removing core but leaving Skin ON.

2. Stir all ingredients together, folding in the marshmallows last.

3. Mix well until all pieces are coated with yogurt.

4. Enjoy!

Amaranth Flatbreads/ Crackers

Prepartion time

20 minutes

Ingredients

- 1 cup amaranth flour (1/4 amaranth flour for rolling)
- 1 Tablespoon arrowroot flour
- 1 tablespoon flaxseed ground or whole (optional)

- 1 teaspoon ground dried chives (any desired herb)
- 2 teaspoons sea salt
- 1/2 cup water
- 2 tablespoons olive

Instructions

1. Preheat oven to 400 degrees.
2. Mix dry ingredients in large bowl together.
3. In separate bowl combine water and oil and beat with a fork.
4. Slowly add water/oil to dry ingredients turning the flour slowly.

5. Mix ingredients until firm ball but not too sticky.

6. Oil flat baking pan and roll out (or pat with hands) small balls of dough until 1/8th inch thick using extra flour to keep from sticking.

7. Place in oven for 3-5 minutes.

8. Remove and flip the flat breads, put them back in the oven for another 3 minutes.

9. They are served well warm or cold, refrigerate any extras.

Turkey Cacciatore #2 with Mushrooms

Prepartion time

6 hours

Ingredients

- 1 turkey breasts, or 4 turkey thighs [or use a BTD compliant substitute]
- olive oil
- spelt flour to coat or rice flour
- 1 chopped large onion
- 1/4 ounces fresh chopped oyster mushroom pieces

- 2 cloves chopped garlic
- 1/4 to 1/2 cup chopped Italian parsley
- 2 Tablespoons fresh oregano or 2 teaspoons dry oregano
- 2 Tablespoons fresh basil or 2 teaspoons dry sweet basil
- 1 teaspoon garlic salt
- 1/2 teaspoon roasted chicory root (optional in place of pepper)
- 2 6-ounce cans of tomato paste [omit A and B secretors]
- 4 fresh juicy chopped tomatoes (or 1 15-ounce stewed tomatoes or tomato sauce)
- 1 teaspoon sugar (optional)

- 1/4 pound fresh green beans
- 1 cup zucchini diced (optional)

Instructions

1. Flour turkey pieces with spelt flour [or use a BTD compliant substitute].

2. Brown turkey in olive oil, do not cook through.

3. Place turkey in the crock pot.

4. Note: While the turkey is browning, season with a mix of sea salt, paprika, sugar, pepper, garlic powder, cumin, turmeric, lemon peel, cayenne, onion and ground mustard (1/2 teaspoon of each previously mixed in a separate bowl).

5. In the fry pan you just used, saute the onion.

6. Add the oyster mushroom pieces.

7. Add garlic, parsley, oregano, basil, garlic salt and roasted chicory root.

8. Add tomatoes, oyster mushrooms and sugar.

9. Saute lightly blending all together.

10. Pour this tomato mixture over the turkey in the crock pot.

11. Add about 1/2 - 1 cup water.

12. Add green beans to the sauce (optional)and lightly stir.

13. Add the zucchini.

14. Cook 4-6 hours until turkey is cooked.

Delicious Zucchini - Pea Meal

Prepartion time

40 minutes

Ingredients

- 3-4 green zucchini
- 1 package of frozen peas(450 gm) or same amount peas
- 6-8 dessert spoon wild rice
- 1 mid-sized onion
- 1 spoon tomato paste or the equivalent tomato
- 1 dessert spoon(not heaping) rock salt

- 1 dessert spoon red pepper or one small hot red pepper, you can also use the Turkish naturally blackened red pepper called isot(esot)
- 1 dessert spoon thyme
- 1 dessert spoon basil
- 1 cup of water
- 1 spoon(not heaping) olive oil
- some jerusalem artichoke, if you like

Instructions

1. Cut the onion to small cubes and pour together with peas and wild rice to a stewpot, turn the heat on.

2. Cut zucchinis to small cubes and pour to the stewpot with the rest of ingredients except olive oil. Add small cut jerusalem artichokes at this step, if you're adding.

3. Let it boil for 10 minutes, you may mix with a wooden or ceramic spoon a few times.(Ceramic is healthiest option for anything that reaches high temperatures while cooking.)

4. Let it cool until you don't feel it hotter than your mouth, then add the olive oil and mix.

5. Now you may serve in small bowls and start to eat.

Spanish Rice/Quinoa

Prepartion time

45 minutes

Ingredients

- 1 pound ground meat. (I use beef or buffalo, but assume that chicken or turkey would work too)
- 2-3 Tablespoons olive oil (I use a lot)
- 1 medium onion, chopped
- 1-2 red and/or green peppers, chopped (I normally use one red, which is a type O beneficial and one green for color)
- 1 carrot, sliced thin (optional for color)
- 1-15 ounce can tomato sauce
- 1-15 ounce can diced tomatoes

- 1 cup rice or quinoa
- 2 teaspoons chili powder, rounded

Instructions

1. Start the rice or quinoa cooking. I use a rice cooker for both.
2. Chop the onion and peppers, and slice the carrot.
3. Brown meat in large covered skillet on medium heat.
4. Drain liquid from the skillet.
5. Add the olive oil, chopped onions and peppers to the skillet and stir to distribute the oil.

6. Cover and let cook until the onions look cooked.

7. Add the 2 cans of tomatoes.

8. Add the chili powder.

9. When vegetables are cooked to your liking add the rice or quinoa to the skillet and stir.

10. Serve.

Basil Pesto

Prepartion time

6 minutes

Ingredients

- enough basil (not packed down) to fill blender
- 2 Tablespoons oil
- 2 lemons or limes, juiced
- 2-5 cloves garlic, pressed
- sea salt to taste
- 1/2-1 cup nuts/seeds

Instructions

1. Put in blender and process until coarse.

2. You may have to stop it and push it down with a rubber spatula.

Basic Dijon-Style Mustard

Prepartion time

6 weeks

Ingredients

- 2 cups (470 ml) dry white wine
- 1 large onion, chopped
- 3 garlic cloves, pressed
- 1 cup (240 ml) dry mustard
- 3 Tablespoons (45 ml) honey [or BTD compliant sweetener]

• 1 Tablespoon (15 ml) olive oil [or BTD compliant oil]

• 2 Teaspoons (10 ml) sea salt

Instructions

1. Combine wine, onion, and garlic in a saucepan.

2. Heat to boiling and simmer 5 minutes.

3. Cool and discard strained solids.

4. Add this liquid to dry mustard, stirring constantly until smooth.

5. Blend in honey, oil, and salt.

6. Return to saucepan (have hankies ready or hold face away from steam) and heat slowly until thickened stirring constantly.

7. Cool.

8. Place in a covered jar.

9. Age in cool, dark place 2 to 8 weeks, depending upon pungency desired, then refrigerate.

Sauteed Grouper

Prepartion time

13 minutes

Ingredients

- 3 Tablespoon olive oil
- 1 to 1.5 pound fresh grouper, trimmed of bones and cut into finger-sized pieces
- 1/2 cup quinoa flour
- salt

Instructions

1. In a large cast iron skillet, heat oil over medium heat.
2. Roll grouper in the flour, shaking off excess.
3. Slip each piece into the hot oil, being careful not to overcrowd the pan.
4. Cook in small batches, adding more oil if necessary.

5. Make sure the oil is very hot before adding the fish.

6. Turn once when nicely browned on one side, then cook another 3 to 4 minutes.

7. Test for doneness.

8. Pat off excess oil on a paper towel and serve.

Banana Carrot Cake

Prepartion time

1 hour 15 minutes

Ingredients

- 1/4 pound butter, chopped [or ghee]

- 1 cup sugar [or brown sugar, maple sugar, agave syrup]
- 1 egg, lightly beaten
- 1 medium carrot, coarsely grated
- 2 over ripe bananas, mashed
- 1-1/2 cups rice flour
- 1 teaspoon baking soda
- 1 teaspoon allspice [B and AB substitute nutmeg]
- 3/4 cup chopped walnuts or pecans
- 1 teaspoon xanthan gum [Best to omit; see Note below]
- 1/4 teaspoon baking powder [Baking Powder Recipe Variations]

[Note: Xanthan gum is not listed in Typebase, but is assumed to be a universal avoid, like other vegetable gums tested so far.]

Instructions

1. Cream butter and sugar in mixer.

2. Add egg beat until combined.

3. Add carrot and banana.

4. Add sifted dry ingredients and nuts, stirring until combined.

5. Spread into prepared 8 inch pan or ring pan.

6. Cook in a moderate oven 180 degrees Celsius [350 degrees Fahrenheit] for about 1 hour or until a skewer comes out clean.

7. Stand in pan for 5 minutes before turning out.

Or:

1. Melt butter and work into the rest of the ingredients.

2. Put into a large microwave ring pan and cook for about 6-1/2 minutes in a 900 Watt microwave oven.

3. Leave in pan as above.

4. Turn out and ice when cold.

5. I use a plain butter icing, or you can sprinkle it with sugar.

6. It is delicious.

Apricot walnut gluten free muffins

Prepartion time

35 minutes

Ingredients

- 1 can of whole apricots in juice
- 2 eggs
- 1 cup of buckwheat flour
- 1 cup of brown rice flour
- 1/4 cup tapioca flour

- 1-1/2 teaspoons of baking powder[baking powder recipes]
- 1-1/2 teaspoons of baking soda
- a pinch of sea salt
- 1/2 cup of brown sugar
- 3 Tablespoons of walnut butter
- raisins

Instructions

1. Mix the eggs and apricots in a food processor. Combine dry ingredients well and then add your liquids.

2. Add raisins last, and taste the mix. If necessary add more brown sugar.

3. Bake in the oven at 350 degrees for 20 - 30 minutes.

Roast Sticky Chicken

Prepartion time

5 hours 20 minutes

Ingredients

- 1-1/3 Tablespoon salt
- 2 teaspoon paprika
- 1 teaspoon onion powder
- 1 teaspoon thyme
- 1/2 teaspoon garlic powder

- 1 Tablespoon sugar
- 1 large roasting chicken
- 1 cup onion, chopped

Instructions

1. In a small bowl, thoroughly combine all the spices.
2. Remove giblets from chicken, clean the cavity well and pat dry with paper towels.
3. Rub the spice mixture into the chicken, both inside and out, making sure it is evenly distributed and down deep into the skin.
4. Place in a resealable plastic bag, seal and refrigerate overnight.

5. When ready to roast chicken, stuff cavity with onions, and place in a shallow baking pan.

6. Roast, uncovered, at 250 degrees for 5 hours (yes, 250 degrees for 5 hours).

7. After the first hour, baste chicken occasionally (every half hour or so) with pan juices.

8. The pan juices will start to caramelize on the bottom of pan and the chicken will turn golden brown.

9. If the chicken contains a pop-up thermometer, ignore it.

10. Let chicken rest about 10 minutes before carving. Freeze all or part in ziplocs after baking.

11. Thaw and reheat, or use meat cold.

Cranberry Apricot Turkey Roll

Prepartion time

12 hours

Ingredients

- 1/4 cup sugar [or BTD compliant variant/substitute]
- 2 Tablespoons arrowroot, don't boil arrowroot
- 3/4 cup apricot jam [BTD compliant variant/substitute]
- 1 cup fresh cranberries, ground or finely chopped

- 2 pound frozen turkey roll or 2 to 2-1/2 pounds partially thawed
- 1 or 2 cups water
- salt and pepper to taste

Instructions

1. In small saucepan, blend sugar and arrowroot.

2. Stir in marmalade and cranberries.

3. Cook and stir until mixture is bubbly and slightly thickened.

4. Place partially thawed turkey roll in slow-cooking pot.

5. Add a cup or two of fresh water.

6. Sprinkle lightly with salt and pepper.

7. Pour sauce over turkey.

8. Cover and cook on low for 9-10 hours.

9. Insert meat thermometer in turkey for the last 2-3 hours.

10. Cover and cook until temperature reaches 185 degrees

11. Slice turkey roll.

12. Serve with vegetables and salad.

Salmon & Rice

Prepartion time

40 minutes

Ingredients

- 1 can of salmon or 1 large salmon steak
- 3 Tablespoons spanish olives
- 1 small onion chopped
- 3 cloves garlic chopped
- olive oil
- 2 small cans tomato sauce
- 2 cups white rice

Instructions

1. In a sauce pan, put 2 cups of rice and 4 cups of water to boil.

2. Once boiling begins, turn down to medium heat and cover for 17 minutes until done.

3. In another fry pan, add 3 Tablespoons olive oil, chopped onion and garlic until clear.

4. Add 2 cans of sauce and 1 half can of water and olives, let simmer for 10 minutes, then add salmon including all juice in can, simmer 10 minutes and serve over rice.

Almond Macaroons

Prepartion time

30 minutes

Ingredients

- 1 roll Odense Almond Paste
- 2/3 cup granulated sugar [or 1/2 amount agave]
- egg whites from 2 large eggs slightly beaten(scant 1/4 cup)
- 1/4 cup chopped almonds (optional)

Instructions

1. Break almond paste into small pieces and place into mixing bowl with the sugar.
2. Mix together with fingers or fork until mixture is crumbly.
3. Add half of the egg whites and mix with electric mixer until a paste begins to form.

4. Add remaining egg whites and continue mixing until a smooth stiff paste is formed.

5. Spoon mixture into walnut-size balls, rolling lightly between palms until smooth.

6. Optional: Press top of cookie into the chopped almonds. Place on greased or non-stick cookie sheet, leaving room for cookies to double in size.

7. Bake at 325 degrees approximately 15-20 minutes until light golden in color. Cookies will be lightly cracked on top.

Green' noodles

Prepartion time

25 minutes

Ingredients

- onions
- garlic
- sea salt
- chopped celery
- diced collard green
- one big bunch of diced parsley
- 2 or 3 strips of turkey bacon
- olive oil
- ghee
- rice noodles
- water

- coriander
- black pepper (a little)[or BTD compliant substitute]

Instructions

1. Saute all of your veggies in the olive oil. Add salt. Stir well and stir often.

2. 5 - 10 minutes later, add 1 cup of water and one package of Thai rice noodles (any rice noodle will do). These Thai noodles cook up in about 6 minutes.

3. Throw in one big tablespoon of ghee (anytime during the cooking process - it's that slight butter flavor I was after.)

4. When noodles are ready, season with more salt, pepper and corainder seed.

5. Sliced gala apples on the side complemented the dish.

Fig Filled Cookies

Prepartion time

25 minutes

Ingredients

- 2 cups dried figs, stems removed, chopped (food processor works very well)
- 1/2 cup sugar (your choice)
- 3/4 cup water

- Juice of 1 lemon
- 1/2 cup butter or ghee
- 1 cup brown sugar
- 2 eggs
- 1 teaspoon vanilla
- 2-1/2 cups BTD flour, might need more if dough is too sticky in bowl
- 1/4 teaspoon soda
- 1/2 teaspoon sea salt

Instructions

1. In a saucepan, combine figs, sugar, water and lemon juice. Cook and stir over medium heat until mixture is thick and jam-like. Cool.

2. In a bowl, combine butter, brown sugar, eggs and vanilla. Stir in flour, soda and salt. Turn dough out onto a heavily floured surface and knead a few times to make a smooth ball.

3. With a floured rolling pin, roll dough out to a 14x12-inch rectangle. Cut dough with a knife into 4 strips, 3-1/2 inches wide and 12 inches long.

4. Spoon filling in a mound down the center of each strip. Using a spatula, turn in side of each strip to enclose filling, press edges together. With a sharp knife, cut each strip into 10 pieces.

5. Place seam-side down on greased baking sheets and bake at 375 Fahrenheit for 10 to 12 minutes, or until cookies are puffed and firm to the touch.

6. Cool on rack and store in an airtight container in a cool dry place.

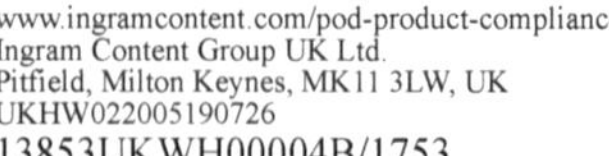
www.ingramcontent.com/pod-product-compliance
Ingram Content Group UK Ltd.
Pitfield, Milton Keynes, MK11 3LW, UK
UKHW022005190726
13853UKWH00004B/1753

9 798537 452218